Atkins Diet

The Complete Guide to
Your Low-Carb Diet
for Rapid Weight Loss and
Healthy Living

Author
Justin Lambert

TABLE OF CONTENTS

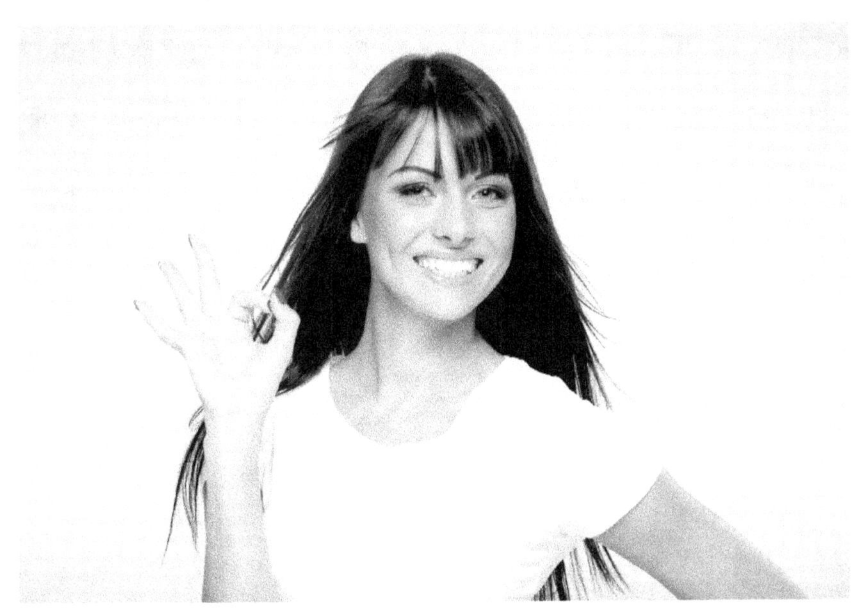

INTRODUCTION

Health.

It is the one thing that affects us every day. The majority of us don't just strive for average health, we want excellent health. We don't want to get sick, nor do we want to live a limited life. Ideally, we want to be the healthiest possible.

Many of us dream of a fit physique, high energy levels, and the feeling that we can conquer anything. However, few of us feel this way. We are often busy, tired, and rushing through meals because we are saddled with busy work schedules, packed family and social lives, and little time for ourselves. What's worse is the lack of awareness about healthy food options that exist for those constantly on the go. Many of us are bombarded with fad diets and numerous experts touting the "best" foods that will help us lose weight.

So how do we choose the right diet for us?

How do we learn which foods to eat?

How do we continuously make choices so they become second nature?

Well there is only one ideal way to live, and that is by maintaining a healthy diet that consists of whole, unprocessed foods and limited refined carbohydrates.

This can be accomplished through the Atkins diet.

It is a way of life that will help you achieve optimum health. You will never look at your quest for fitness, weight loss, and optimum health as drudgery or sacrifice. Your energy levels and renewed health will be all the motivation you'll need. The Atkins

Diet can change everything.

In this book, we will discuss the core principles of the Atkins Diet, in addition to learning more about Dr. Robert Atkins and his research history. This book will also cover the difference between other ineffective low carbohydrate diets and the Atkins Diet. Additionally, we will discuss why the science of the Atkins Diet still works, while others don't. This book will serve as a how-to guide. It will show you how to prepare for the Atkins Diet, sample menus, and how to understand that the Atkins Diet is not a fleeting trend, but a way of life.

By the instruction, research, and data outlined here, the Atkins Diet will show you how to avoid mistakes, commit completely, and acquire the lifestyle you've always wanted.

So, let's begin!

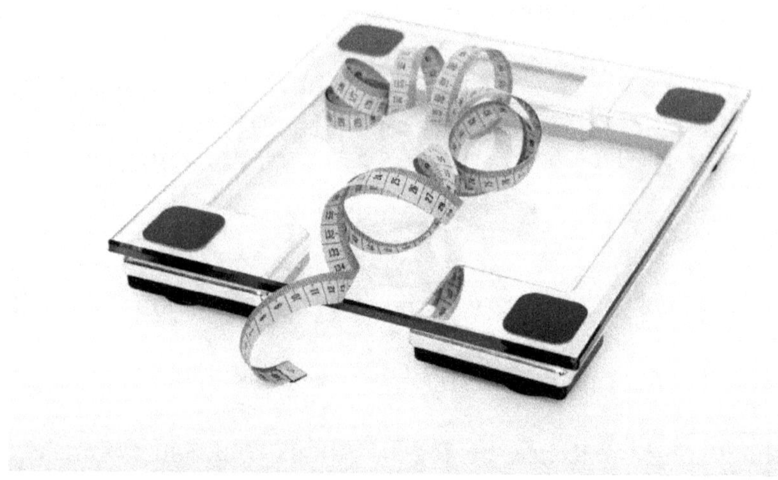

WHAT IS THE ATKINS DIET?

The Atkins Diet is a nutritional plan created by Dr. Robert C. Atkins. His patient work over the years left him questioning why a growing number of people were unfit and unhealthy despite medical advances, a wide availability of fresh food, and helpful dietary guidelines that were accessible to all people. He wanted to understand the mistakes people were making while providing a clear-cut way to instruct people on how to nourish themselves while helping them to lose weight and improve their health for the long-term.

Dr. Robert Atkins worked as a cardiologist and as an internist (internal medicine). Due to the large number of patients he saw with declining health issues, he studied his patients and created the Atkins nutritional approach in the 1970's as a response to his patients' metabolic disorders. He published his first book about the Atkins nutritional approach in 1972. Even though it had initial success and gained widespread popularity, it continues to differ from other diets that have come and gone. The Atkins Diet is still globally known today for a good reason: it works.

The Atkins Diet provides scientifically tested suggestions for what to eat and how to change your metabolic functioning in order to stay fit. The diet centers around minimal, low-carbohydrates, along with the consumption of healthy fats and protein. This will provide individuals with a full feeling that lasts, leading to permanent physical change and renewed health.

Furthermore, the Atkins Diet states that low-fat and low-calorie fad diets fail so often because individuals are not properly nourished. As a result, they experience severe hunger pangs and other physical triggers that make them unable to sustain those harsh restrictions and eating patterns. This extreme deprivation and calorie counting leads to "yo-yo dieting," bingeing, and other unsafe eating patterns. While the dieter may lose the weight initially, they gain it back, while sometimes adding additional weight on. Fad diets do not work and are dangerous. They do not provide a lifestyle change, nor do they provide a healthy short-term solution.

The Atkins Diet focuses on health by sufficiently nourishing the body. Individuals who begin the Atkins Diet will not be hungry. They will feel full and alert, while they gradually lose weight. This diet also leads to a steady, healthy weight for their body, along with eating patterns that can be followed for life.

The Atkins Diet strongly discourages the consumption of sugar and useless, refined carbohydrates. This absence of processed carbohydrates (for example, bread or cookies) will eliminate midday crashing and overall fatigue. As a result, the rushed, over-eating patterns of consuming easiest available food option (usually sleep inducing fast food) will vanish as well. Once the tiredness is gone, energy levels will also rise. Snacking will be minimal, if needed at all. Individuals will begin to look for only whole proteins and healthy options. The Atkins Diet will become a way of life.

The Atkins Diet encourages the steady consumption of whole foods, while eliminating junk food or fast food entirely. This may seem impossible for you, but eventually the high salt and sugar found in those foods will become undesirable. Especially, in comparison to the healthy and filling proteins found in lean meats and fish, for example.

The Atkins Diet challenges the standard (and harmful) Northern American diet that we have all come to know and adopt. Through common sense principles of eating whole foods like vegetables, healthy fats (like olive oil and nuts), and protein, like chicken, fish, or eggs, all individuals trying the Atkins Diet will increase their health and energy, create a healthy metabolism, while greatly decreasing the possibility of chronic disease, like diabetes, hypertension, heart disease, or worse.

One of the main principles of the Atkins diet, is to limit or eradicate the existence of refined carbohydrates in the diet. This is a central and essential component. This diet does not focus on watching calorie intake, but rather integrating healthy foods that make sense. The body is not capable of handling the consumption of heavy carbohydrate foods (which provide no nutrients or fuel), while losing weight or maintaining a healthy and fit physique. Additionally, the possibility of losing weight and keeping weight off while consuming, low-fat foods (which are often processed and refined carbohydrates), is impossible.

Principles of the Atkins diet will focus on changing metabolic disruptions in your body, reducing your dependency on high carbohydrate, nutrient deficient foods. You will not be counting calories, but instead begin to focus on whole proteins, fresh vegetables, and healthy fats as a way to fuel your body and feel like you can accomplish anything during the day without feeling low. As you will learn, healthy fats and lean protein are crucial for a nourished body.

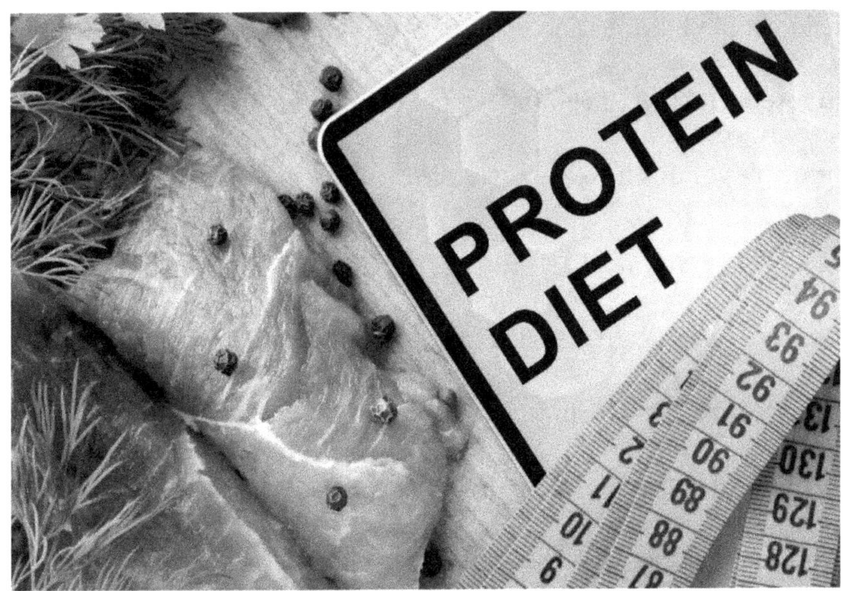

THE HISTORY OF THE ATKINS DIET

The Atkins Diet was originally known as the Atkins nutritional approach when it was first introduced. In these early years, fad diets were not as widespread as they are today. Calling it a nutritional approach truly exemplified what it was—an approach that provides nutrition and can change people's lives.

Dr. Robert C. Atkins began this nutritional approach based on a medical research paper he read in 1958. In his earliest books in the 1970's which introduced his diet said that the differentiating factor between the Atkins Diet and others is that the Atkins Diet will help people burn fat and consequently calories. People will be able to lose weight and keep the weight off, if they understood the basic principles of this low-carbohydrate plan.

The Atkins Diet focuses on an incorrect element in the standard American diet and its recommended food servings. For example, the Food Guide Pyramid suggests six to eleven servings per day of refined carbohydrates like bread, pasta, cereal, or rice, while stating that only three to five servings of vegetables and only two to three servings of proteins are needed in a person's diet. Dr. Atkins challenged this older belief, based on the failing health and increased weight levels of the patients he saw every day.

According to his book, *Dr. Atkins' New Diet Revolution*, he says that the trouble began when industry titans, government officials, and lobbyists started incorrectly influencing the public. There was a time where sugar was not discouraged much as it should have been. Low fat messages were wrongly advocated in the 1980's and 1990's and it lead to the disastrous health of the majority of people today. Food companies responded to these trends by marketing fast, pre-packaged, and processed foods with "low-fat" or "fat-free," while adding addictive sugar or sugar substitute properties.

Prior to the Atkins Diet's introduction, many people assumed that wheat portions were an essential part of a healthy diet and that fats that came from olive oil or butter for example were the food elements to eliminate. This is because people thought a diet with any fat at all was bad. However, studies have shown how incorrect these principles were and are. Carbohydrates like bread and pasta offer no nutritional value. Healthy fats from protein like fish, nuts, or olive oil, can provide essential nutrients, leaving people feeling nourished and full of energy for the entire day.

Historically, Dr. Atkins was the first diet researcher to make these claims. He stated that a low-carb diet makes positive, fat burning changes to a person's metabolism. The Atkins Diet limits carbohydrates that do not provide energy or value. Many carbohydrates can negatively change a person's blood sugar level, causing severe problems later on down the road.

Additionally, Dr. Atkins proposed that a diet with servings of carbohydrates that equal or outdo servings of protein lead to hunger. This is why a low-fat diet (which essentially means high carbohydrates) does not work. People may lose weight quickly at first, but their hunger will cause problems like overeating. The body is also not designed to break down and digest carbohydrates as easily as proteins or fiber (found in vegetables).

In his books, he reiterates that a healthy, long-term, sustainable diet needs to possess healthy fats, protein, and fiber as its core components. Only then can people begin to lose weight and keep it off.

The history of the Atkins Diet stems from Dr. Atkins examination of sugar levels hidden in carbohydrates. Based on his work with patients and his examination of previously (and incorrectly) established government approved food serving guidelines, he determined that carbohydrates needed to be eliminated in order to promote health and increase weight loss.

In the Atkins nutritional approach, Dr. Atkins diet plan proposals are the still the same as the core principles of the diet now.

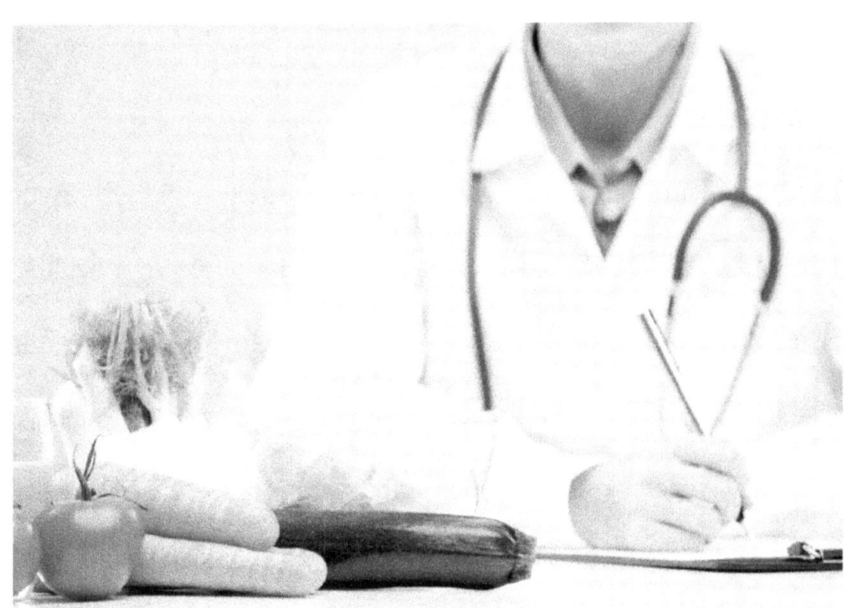

THE DIFFERENCE BETWEEN THE ATKINS DIET
AND OTHER LOW-CARB DIETS

The reason why the Atkins Diet has lasted is simply because it is realistic, does not leave people hungry, and does not center around deprivation.

Other low-carb diets have principles that mirror the essential components of the Atkins Diet, but may take on a more Mediterranean focus by including more fish and olive oil as daily food requirements.

In other variations of low-carb diets, people choose to cut all refined and processed carbs from their diets and consume only animal proteins, spices (for flavor), and related fats like oil. With zero carbs consumed, drastic weight loss and a return to a healthy metabolism results. However, this variation of a low-carb diet has an absence of essential vitamins and nutrient rich properties found in fruits and vegetables. For people who were obese or had serious health issues, the quick and immediate elimination of all carbs may be too drastic. This may result in overeating at a later time. A gradual lessening of all refined carbohydrates is ideal. This will prevent yo-yo dieting and can better result in lasting change.

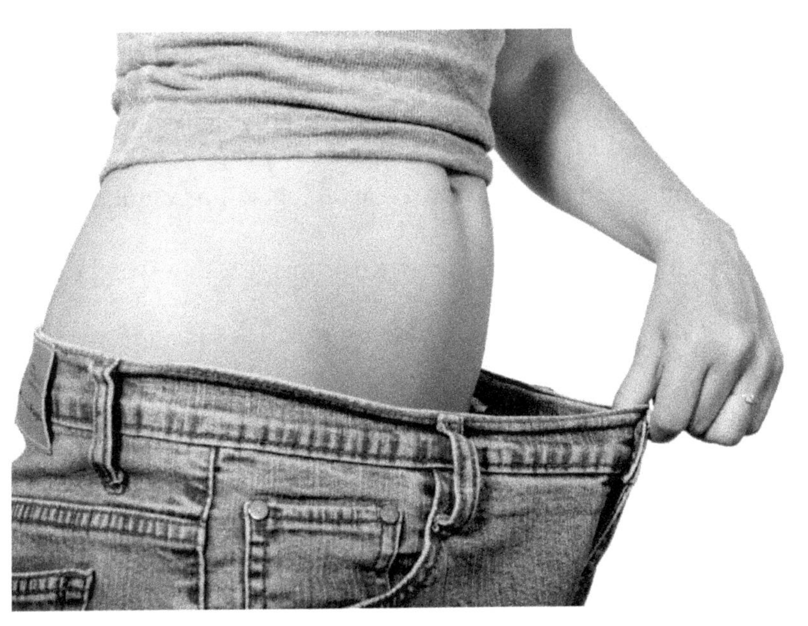

THE SCIENCE BEHIND THE ATKINS DIET: WHY IT WORKS

The Atkins Diet works and has lasted in popular culture's realm because of the word-of mouth results and its practical principles. The science behind the Atkins diet focuses on carbohydrates and addictive sugar and flour.

Understanding the dangers of excessive sugar is an important component for losing weight, keeping it off, and maintaining high levels of above average health. High blood sugar levels are severely problematic if sustained, because the body cannot digest processed foods (like pasta), that are not found in nature. A pasta tree does not exist! And your body is a natural entity. It will have a difficult time breaking down something so unnatural, factory created, and highly processed. Over time, this leads to weight gain and a sometimes, permanent metabolic change. It will become difficult to not only lose the weight, but it will be hard to fight off the cravings caused by the addictive flavors and properties found in starchy, non-nutritional food, like pasta, cookies, or cereal.

Dr. Atkins' extensive patient work and research through the years led him to examine insulin and its dangerous levels in his patients. Based on this, he proposed that the carbohydrates people were consuming in a standard American diet were (and still are) very harmful. This is because it produces high levels of glucose in people.

The types of carbohydrates consumed will definitely have an effect on blood sugar levels. This can be positive or negative. In a standard Northern American diet, foods filled with flour and processed, refined sugar properties are common. There is high fructose corn syrup in almost everything. From store bought salad dressings to pre-packaged sandwiches and cookies, refined sugar and flour is everywhere.

Dr. Atkins centered the development of this diet in part on the science and examination of rising blood sugar levels in people. Insulin brings glucose through your blood and moves it until it hits your cells. However, as sugar levels rise, it cannot be converted into energy due to the refined nature of the carbohydrates. So, your body stores that unneeded, excess glucose as fat. This is exemplified physically through visible weight gain and physical transformations like: beer bellies, "love handles", and cellulite pockets on the belly, hips, buttocks, thighs, and other parts of the leg region.

Excess glucose from refined carbohydrates produces excess fat. And while, you may have mistakenly believed that a low-fat diet is needed, you were misguided. The main culprit in preventable diseases like heart disease, stroke, and diabetes is sugar.

High levels of carbohydrate consumption, which is common today and has been for decades, results in high blood sugar levels. When insulin is overproduced, energy is not properly converted. This leads to common experiences that you may have felt like midday sleepiness, the inability to focus at school or work, or other ailments that affect your ability to be productive or fully present during the day.

Carbohydrate food staples like mashed potatoes, sugar, cream, or French fries, are common in Northern American diets. The dangerous downside is that they can quickly convert to high levels of glucose. And based on the food pyramid, people are following its guidelines, even though they are harmful for them. Higher consumption levels of vegetables and nutrient rich proteins are better for blood sugar levels and your overall health.

An overweight or obese person has already experienced negative changes to their metabolism. Their insulin ability may not be effective and so their body starts storing excess glucose, which is fat. When insulin becomes excessive it leads to severe health risks like obesity. This level of insulin can cause a person to have no energy, excessive fat, and physical limitations.

Another result is that you will need more and more refined carbohydrates. Your body will become used to those foods and it will be what you crave. This is due to metabolic changes, physical routines, and the addictive chemical properties found in refined carbohydrates, processed food and desserts, and nearly all packaged food items that fill the grocery store aisles today.

In his scientific research findings, Dr. Atkins talks about the health issues that result from improper insulin levels. According to his book, Dr. Atkins states numerous times that the process of excess blood glucose will lead to an overproduction of what your body needs. In many people, especially those who consume unnatural, processed carbohydrates, may have a higher chance of developing hyperinsulinism and consequently diabetes. Obesity, breast cancer, and heart disease (which is a leading killer) are completely preventable through maintaining a healthy weight and limiting refined carbohydrate ridden foods.

The scientific connection between life threatening illnesses and insulin abnormalities is a trend that Dr. Atkins noticed was rising. Now diabetes and other related diseases are a pervasive part of our societies. This is due to multiple factors like an incorrect food servings suggestion guide as well as the introduction and spread of fast food outlets and chains.

Science data shows that cardiovascular diseases are definitely connected to insulin resistance and excessive glucose in the blood and body. Heart disease is the leading cause of death. For most people, this is entirely preventable through lifestyle and dietary changes. These dietary changes need to be lasting, effective, and rational. And the Atkins' Diet will help you make these vital changes in your life. The best course of action for your mind, body, and overall health can be achieved through the healthy ways of the Atkins Diet.

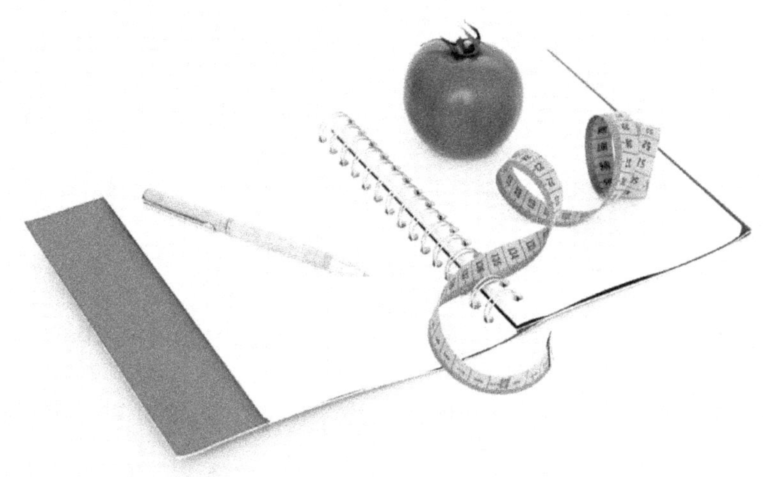

HOW TO PREPARE FOR THE ATKINS DIET

The first way to prepare for the Atkins Diet (aside from reading this starter guide of course!) is to understand that continued consumption of excessive refined carbohydrates will make it difficult to lose weight. If you crave them after a long day of work, late at night, or when you are going through a stressful period, it is best not to have them in the house. There is no nutritional value in flour or sugar. Do not buy these food products. Do not keep them in your house. You are one step closer to fully adopting the Atkins

Diet, by eradicating your home access to carbohydrates.

Secondly, you need to understand that fad diets that include low-fat suggestions are not good for you and do not align with the Atkins Diet in any way. Fat won't cause abnormalities and disruptions to your glucose or insulin. Rather, it will help you feel full when you consume whole, healthy proteins. On the Atkins Diet, you will be eating the right amounts and you won't be hungry throughout the day like when you consume refined carbohydrates. For example, healthy fats from fish will nourish your body with omega-3 and other fatty acids. These properties can help stave off certain diseases when consumed in alignment with the complete Atkins Diet.

You may think that you do not have the willpower to resist certain foods or that you do not have the strength to skip snacking, which was most likely part of your old (unhealthy) routine. But be prepared for the positive changes! Once you start and stick with the Atkins Diet, you will only eat full meals full or nutrient rich foods. Your body will use your fat and burn it. You will realize that you won't be hungry because your food is being properly allocated where it is needed…as energetic fuel.

Be prepared to stop counting calories. The Atkins Diet can help you lose weight and improve your health by guiding with you with food choices that are healthy and filling. Counting calories or total deprivation is not a sustainable eating plan or way of life. The Atkins Diet is.

If you adopt the Atkins Diet be prepared to choose certain food groups. This is needed because as you will learn and as we will discuss later on in this guide, natural, unprocessed carbohydrates may be allowed to be part of your diet. It is crucial to prepare and understand the differentiating factors between certain food groups that the Atkins Diet encourages you to have. You also have to be prepared to pay attention to your body and what it responds to.

For instance, fiber can be considered a carbohydrate in some cases. And it can be a part of your diet, because it is good for you. Fiber absorbs toxic elements in the body, acts as a natural diuretic, improves the immune system, and rids the body of bad cholesterol, to name a few. Fiber can be found in fruits, vegetables, nuts, and unprocessed grains. At the start of the Atkins Diet, many encourage the consumption of vegetables only, until you are used to eating them regularly. Then, the introduction of other sources of fiber will be helpful to give yourself a diet that is well rounded and pleasing.

The Atkins Diet was created and exists as a form of natural healthcare, renewal, and change. However, if you are overweight, have suffered from serious health problems (or are still suffering from them), or are obese, it is important to always consult a doctor prior to beginning this nutritional approach.

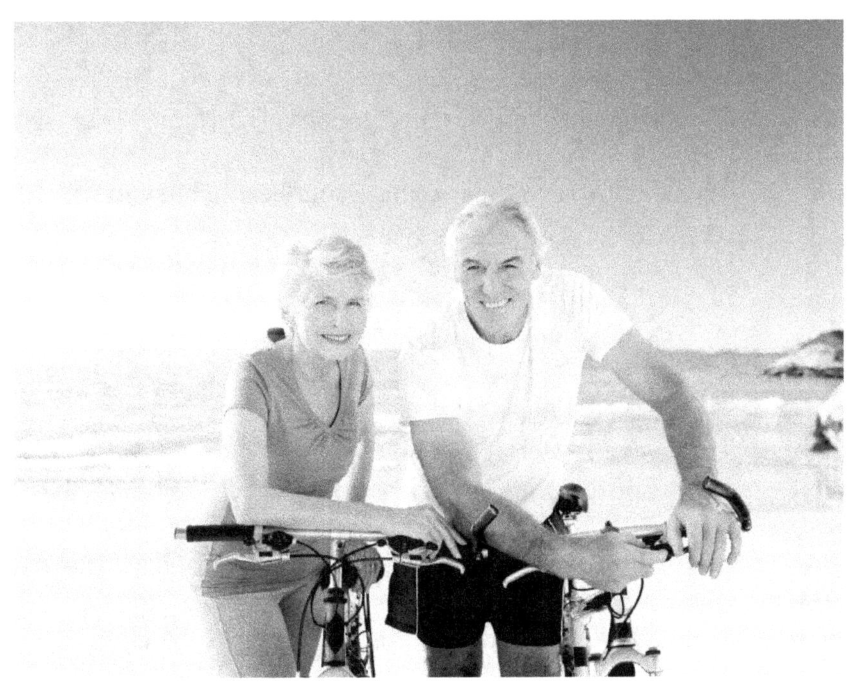

MEDICAL AWARENESS

For those who are starting this diet as a response to their current poor state of health or physical limitations, there is much to be proud of. You have made a decision. You have done your research. You have decided that the Atkins Diet sounds like rational and realistic possibility for you to adopt, in order to change. However, there are still medical facets to consider in relation to your current state of health or to any illnesses you may be suffering from.

- It is important to continue taking any diabetes injections or heart medications. The Atkins' Diet can help you begin to change your health, but you still need to be aware of your current health issues and address those problems by taking your prescribed medication.

- Consult your physician and let him or her know that you are starting the Atkins' Diet. If they have any additional instructions about the diet or your medication, follow their advice. Listen to their guidance. They will be proud of you for taking a proactive first step towards change. Additionally, any doctor will tell you that cutting refined sugar in carbohydrates is a great step.

- While consulting your physician you should also get a complete and thorough physical, along with any other applicable tests, as well as blood work. Once you have implemented the Atkins Diet in your life, looking back at your physical will be a starting point.

You will proudly be able to see how far you've come.

- After you have committed and begun the Atkins Diet, you and your doctor will have to pay close attention to any effects that your medication has your blood sugar levels decreasing due to the Atkins Diet. The quantity or dosage may need to change, based on their decision.

- Communicate closely and regularly with your medical doctor, especially if you currently have or did suffer from any physical health disease.

ADVANTAGES OF THE ATKINS DIET

The Atkins Diet is still around years after Dr. Atkins first presented his research and wrote several best-selling books, because the Atkins Diet provides sustainable results and a healthy lifestyle change. Plain and simple.

While the thought of giving up your previous diet of delicious tasting (unhealthy) snacks and foods may seem daunting, it is important to remember the advantages of the Atkins Diet. For one, the Atkins Diet results in positive metabolic change, which will allow you to burn fat, lose weight, and feel good about yourself. It is a realistic change that can be a permanent part of your life.

The Atkins Diet will stabilize your blood sugar. This is crucial in order to have fewer cravings and binges. It is incredibly beneficial to only consume healthy spaced out meals at appropriate times. The Atkins Diet principles will help you eliminate useless snacking throughout the day.

Some of the advantages to the Atkins Diet are the health benefits. The foods that this diet encourages are incredibly nutrient rich, natural, and unprocessed. Lean meat, fish, eggs, and whole vegetables, to name a few, energize the body. Millions of years ago, people ate the same natural foods from the ground and sea, and had no presence of the modern heart diseases of today.

The Atkins Diet will give health and energy advantages in your life. You will not be eating empty calories but rather, satisfying, tasty food. It may be a diet plan, but it is not a deprivation filled diet. There are many advantages and a lot to look forward too. Your new body, your new mind, and your new outlook are steps away. Keep reading to learn more about what's coming up.

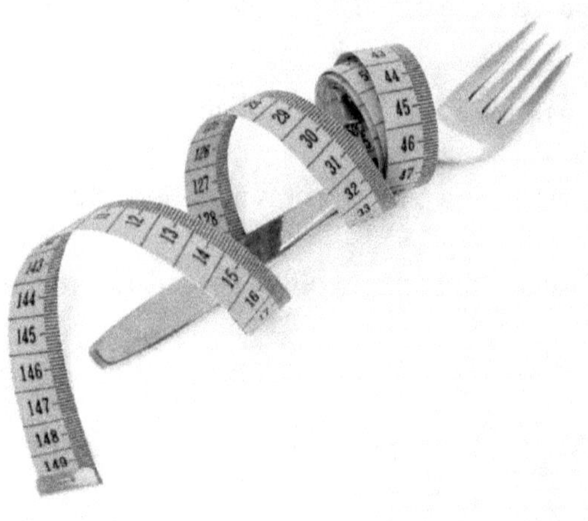

STARTING THE ATKINS DIET – THE FOUR PHASES

Phase 1 – The Induction

The Atkins Diet begins with The Induction phase. This starting point was created to help you change your body's metabolic functioning to become a healthy fat burning machine. This first phase will also help you get rid of cravings and poor eating choices and stabilize your blood sugar.

However, you must understand that the Induction phase is not permanent. It will last no more than two weeks (fourteen days).

After this time, your body will have made noticeable strides in changing your health for the better.

- In the Induction phase, you will eat three typical sized meals or four (or five) smaller meals per day.

- During your awake, daytime hours, do not go more than six hours without eating either a regular meal or a smaller meal.

- You will eat whole proteins and healthy fats from lean meats (for example: chicken or red meat), fish, or eggs.

- Healthy, unprocessed fats found in olive oil, vegetable oil, or butter are allowed to add flavor or to cook protein items with.

- Do not consume more than three cups (or twenty grams) of vegetable carbohydrates per day.

- Absolutely no refined or processed carbohydrates. This includes any junk food, pasta, bread, other grains, fruit, potatoes, nuts, or seeds.

- Fiber rich foods that offer both carbohydrates and protein servings, like beans are not allowed during the induction phase.

- Avoid foods or drinks that are unnaturally sweetened.

- Absolutely no caffeine during this phase. This includes coffee, tea, and especially no unhealthy soft drinks! No soda allowed ever!

- Drink generous amounts of water throughout the day to help control hunger and to help your body adjust.

- Do not be fooled by "sugar free" labels. Examine the contents on the back and check. You are now aware of what it takes to commit to a diet plan.

Phase 2 – Ongoing Weight Loss (OWL)

When you begin phase 2, you may add 5 more grams to your diet per day. So, you may consume a total of 25 grams of carbohydrates. Adding vegetables is the healthiest and most filling way to go in phase 2. After every successful week, you may increase your carbohydrate intake by 5 grams.

During this phase, you may add variety to your carbohydrate intake. You may include certain fruits, nuts, and seeds. Certain aged cheeses are also allowed in small 5 ounce quantities. This phase is about understanding limited and regulated carbohydrate consumption. However, it is important to be aware that nuts and seeds can be difficult to eat only a few of. Be careful.

Phase 3 – Pre-Maintenance

At this point, your healthy eating habits have produced results. You have lost significant weight and are getting closer to your target every day. You committed to a plan to change and it has worked!

In this phase, you can add 10 more grams to your diet each week. You may integrate more healthy food options into your diet, like a wider selection of fruits for example. However, you can only increase your carbohydrate gram intake by 10, if you continue to steadily lose weight.

Towards the end of this phase you can also increase your carb intake up to 20 grams two or three times per week. This can only occur if you are on track with your weight and still have high energy levels. Additionally, other items like potatoes, fruit, or even a glass of dry wine may be included in your new diet. However, if certain fruits or wine triggers sugar cravings or an increase in appetite, it is best to slowly decrease your carbohydrate allowance and start later when you feel you have it under control.

This phase is important because it is the time to progress

carefully. Do not try to increase your carbohydrate intake too fast or

lose too much weight during this third phase. Slow is the word to

remember during this time.

Phase 4 – Lifetime Maintenance

Congratulations! You have come so far. There is much to be proud of. These kind thoughts will help you power your way through. In this phase, you realize that this way of eating is for life. You can stay healthy and fit, you can have tons of energy, and you do not need those useless empty calories. You know what your body can handle, especially in terms of carbohydrate offerings.

This last phase sometimes mirrors phase 2 (OWL). Understand your body and how many grams of carbohydrates is suitable. Your body may be able to handle starchy carbohydrates like potatoes, or it may not. Recognize which fruits are a trigger for cravings and eliminate them. Continue to eat whole, unrefined carbohydrates. Unprocessed fruits and vegetables are ideal. Implement a fitness routine. Realize that this renewed health is yours.

This phase is also about excitement and acceptance. At this phase, make sure to keep your fridge and freezer stocked with delicious proteins and vegetables. Learning new, healthy recipes and developing meals you like and look forward to very is important. By now you will recognize how many carb grams is ideal for you and what healthy options (vegetables, fruits, grains) are preferable. Now, it is all about choice.

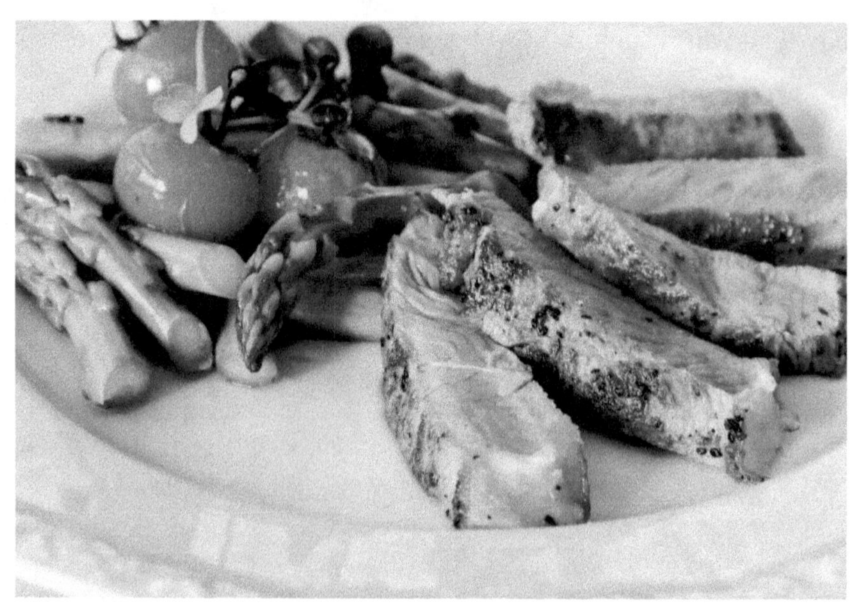

WHAT TO EAT AND WHAT TO AVOID ON THE ATKINS DIET

The Atkins Diet is a nutritional approach. And because all individuals are different in physical and interior makeup, there may be variances in your approach to what works for you, regarding your food selection and count. The most important thing to remember is that you should feel nourished and energized, not grumpy and severely starving. If you do take the Atkins Diet to an extreme degree because you want to lose more than one pound a day, you may put yourself in danger. This is not something that is advised by any medical professional or Dr. Atkins' principles. If you do lose more than one pound a day, it is most likely certain that you will gain it back, which is often the result with other fad diets.

Your metabolic system needs to adjust to the Atkins nutritional approach, slowly and carefully. This is especially true if you have been suffering from health problems and have been consuming a nutrient deficient diet. The Atkins Diet principles strongly advise that you do not lose more than one pound a day. There are a few exceptions. People who are described as overweight or obese by their doctors may lose more than one pound during the earliest stages, but not for the entirety of the Atkins Diet.

Ultimately, the Atkins nutritional approach should serve as strict guidelines. If you follow them you will succeed in restoring your health. We'll begin by discussing specifics about what to eat and what to avoid during the Atkins Diet and for your new life.

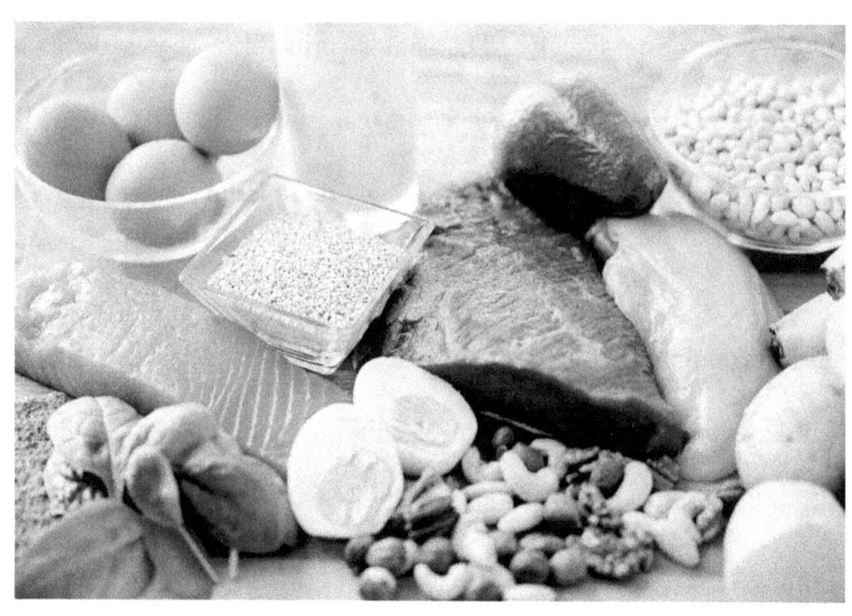

FOODS YOU MAY EAT (ESPECIALLY DURING THE INDUCTION PHASE):

- Generous amounts of lean proteins will become paramount during your three meals (or four smaller meals) in this phase and all phases of the Atkins Diet.

- Specifically, you may eat meats like chicken, beef, pork, veal, lamb, turkey, duck, and natural seafood (try to avoid imitation shellfish). However, do not overeat. It is best to eat until you are satisfied, but never overly stuffed.

- No more than two and a half cups of vegetables like mushrooms, radishes, peppers, cucumbers, celery, artichokes, asparagus, broccoli, cauliflower, eggplant, onion, squash, tomato, okra, pumpkin, zucchini, olives, and all green leafy vegetables are permitted.

- Oils and healthy fats like olive oil, mayonnaise, and butter are allowed.

- Any spices and or herbs to add flavor to meats are allowed. No sugar. Be extra cautious and check the labels of all herbs to be sure.

- Aim for eight ounces of water a day. Lemon and lime are excellent supplements to your daily water consumption.

- Decaffeinated teas and coffee are permitted. It is best to drink them black and with no additives. If this is too difficult of an adjustment, two tablespoons of cream are acceptable.

- No more than four ounces of aged cheeses per day.

- Never exceed more than 20 grams of carbohydrates. This is crucial during the Induction phase.

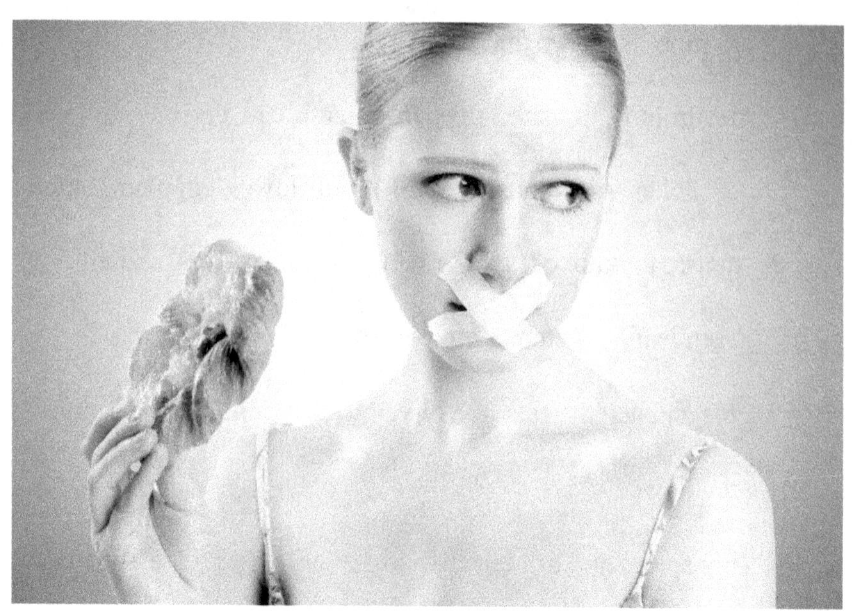

FOODS TO AVOID (PARTICULARLY DURING THE INDUCTION PHASE):

- You should completely avoid rice, all grains, potatoes, pasta, pizza, bread, crackers, cereals, beans, legumes, and fruit.

- Avoid high-sugar or starchy vegetables like corn, beets, carrots, potatoes, yams, peas, and parsnips.

- Absolutely no cottage cheese or cream cheese. Their carbohydrate level is too high.

- Avoid nuts and seeds.

- Absolutely no alcohol.

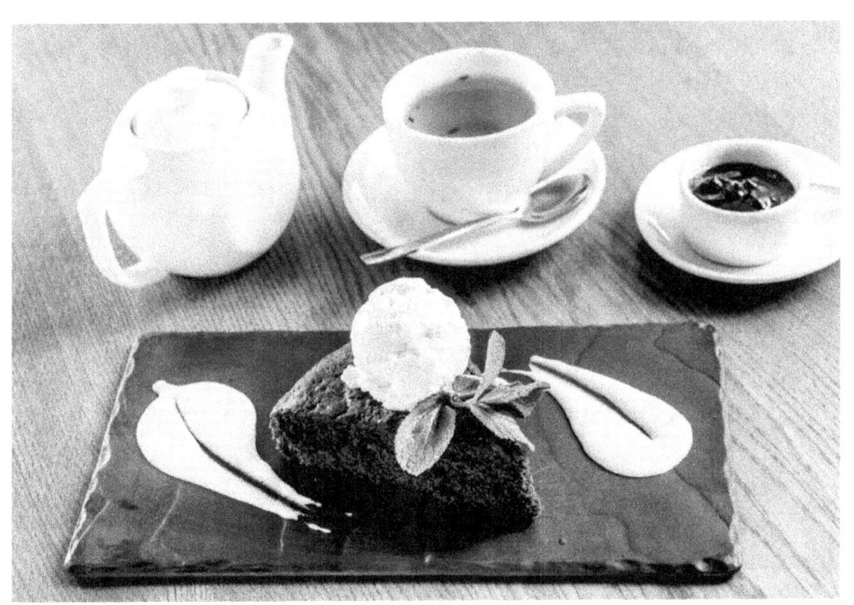

FOODS TO ALWAYS AVOID:

- Avoid all sugars.

- Absolutely no sweetened condiments like store made salad dressings, ketchup, or barbeque sauce.

- Avoid artificially sweetened drinks or foods of any kinds (examples: sodas, sweetened iced teas, or jello).

- Absolutely no processed carbohydrates, junk food, or processed food or drink items of any kind. This includes sodas, chips, cookies, or pies. If you know it is not healthy and is considered junk food, do not eat it.

Processed sugar, junk food, sodas, and useless carbohydrates are unhealthy and toxic. These foods should always be avoided. They are now part of your *past* life. It is time to positively look forward at your new body, health, and new life that awaits. Congratulate yourself for taking the positive steps to have found the Atkins Diet and to be able to fully commit to the outline above. Fruits, legumes, corn, and nuts are foods that may be gradually integrated into your diet during later phases, as mentioned in phase 3 and 4. However, the lists above emphasize whole, natural, and unprocessed foods. These are the food guidelines that will give you renewed health now and for the rest of your life.

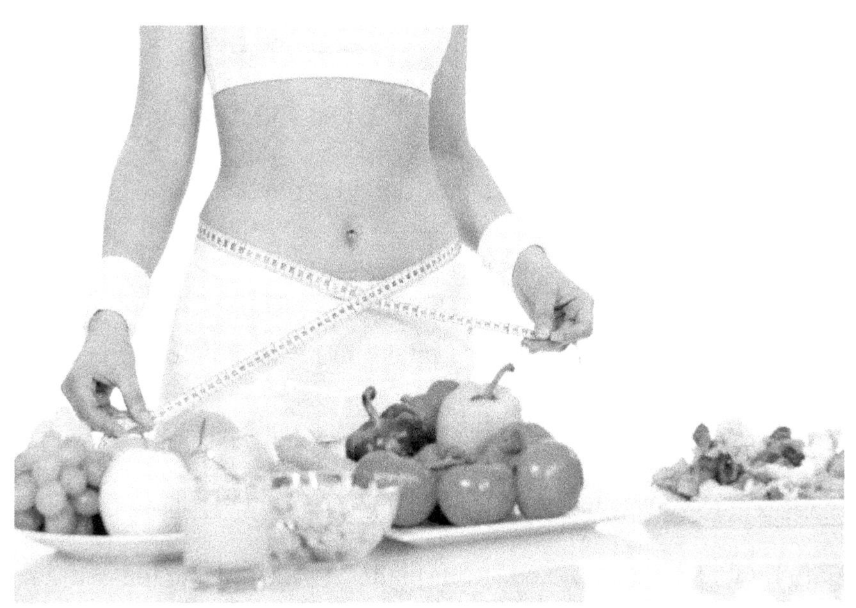

MONITORING CARBOHYDRATE INTAKE

One way to monitor carbohydrate intake is to pay close attention to the food label. On the ingredients list, not all carbohydrates are good and not all are bad. But the way to figure out the carbohydrates that the Atkins Diet wants you to pay attention to is to minus the grams listed under the dietary fiber from the total number of carbohydrate grams.

Check your serving sizes. This can also be found on the label. Just because a food portion says twenty calories does not mean that's all it has. The serving size might be five. So, the actual calorie count for that food portion would be 100. Understand where those calories come from. Are they coming from sources of fuel and energy or are they coming from excess sugar?

Monitoring carbohydrate intake in restaurants may be more challenging. Some general rules would be to make sure that the food items you choose are unprocessed carbohydrates. Choose simple starters like a cheese and fruit platter (if you have passed the induction phase), or olives, or a sample vegetable platter. Avoid all bread. If your server has not brought out the bread basket, please ask that they do not, that way it is easier to avoid temptation.

For your main courses, ways to monitor your carbohydrate intake is to avoid proteins that are fried with breading or additives. Choose a meat protein like lobster, lamb, or fish that is baked, if possible. Choose a small solo side of vegetables like spinach or mushrooms. Asked what they are cooked in and if there are any bread or grain additives. Your waiter or waitress should be familiar with these staples. And it never hurts to ask.

When you are travelling as so many people do today,

monitoring your carbohydrate intake can be difficult, but it is

certainly not impossible. One way to avoid falling off your diet

pathway is to pack food at home. If it is a day trip, this is a

beneficial method for your diet, your health, and your wallet!

Airport or train station food is expensive. Pack raw veggies, hard

boiled eggs, pre-sliced cold cut turkey, and cubed cheese for a

breakfast, lunch, or snack option while you're traveling. Airports

allow food to be brought on flights, so there is no excuse why you

cannot adhere to the Atkins Diet on the road. Give yourself plenty of

time to look for healthy options, if you want to have a more filling,

sit-down meal at the airport or train station before boarding. Order

dinner sized portions of cooked chicken, beef, or fish. Ask them to

hold the sides of potatoes or whatever else it comes with. This is

ideal. It is also one less thing for the chef or serving crew to have to

prepare.

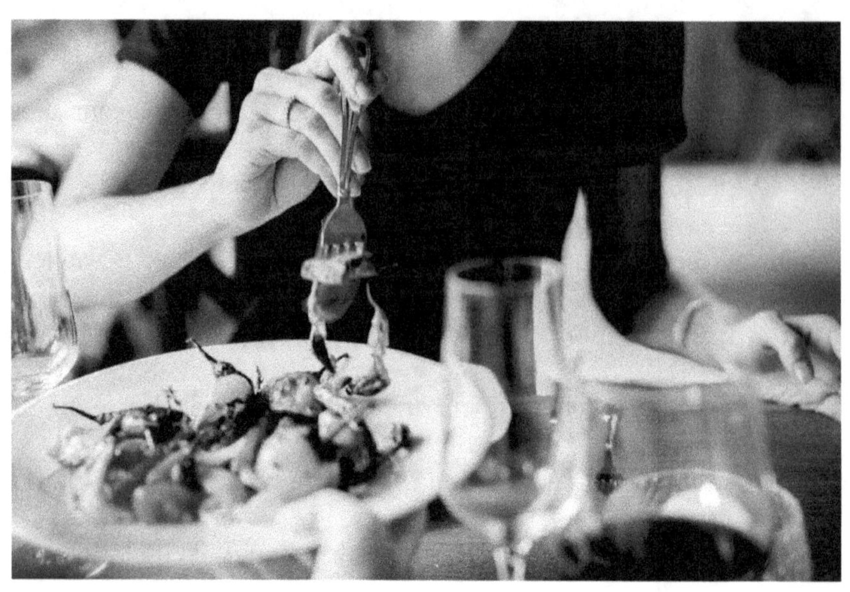

ATKINS DIET TIPS FOR SPECIAL CIRCUMSTANCES

While this starter guide outlines the core elements and examples of the Atkins Diet, committing to the Atkins Diet may be difficult for two main reasons: negative influences and willpower.

Telling your medical doctor about your Atkins Diet plans is necessary, but it is also important to tell the people closest to you in your life. Your spouse, significant other, friends, roommates, children, and family should all know, especially if they live with you.

A tip for sticking to the Atkins Diet are to separate your food items. If you are a parent, it might benefit the entire family to not allow any processed and refined carbohydrates in the house any longer. However, with just a significant other or roommate, put your foods, condiments, and drinks in a separate, far place like a cupboard far from theirs or a low drawer seldom used in the fridge. Whatever they choose to eat is their choice. However, it will limit temptation if you never see those other foods that you used to consume from your past life and from your former self. Label your food drawers in the fridge or pantry. Organize them. Make your new diet look enticing in every way. Train yourself not to look into your roommate's cupboards or section of the pantry.

If there are still obstacles, have them read this starter guide. Get them to understand the health consequences that await if you don't start to change. Talk to them openly and kindly. Get them to understand that this is important to you and is not just a temporary diet, but a complete lifestyle change. If they are responsive and seem to understand, encourage them to start the diet as well. You can act as a support system for one another.

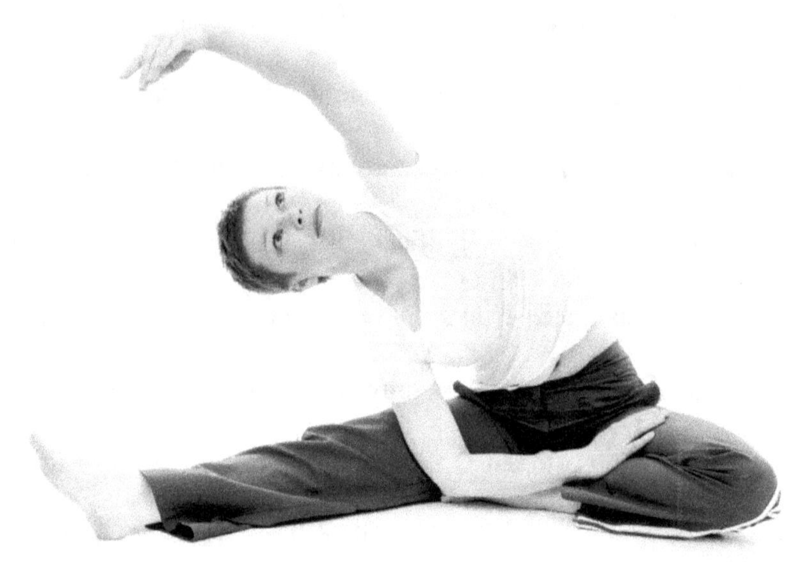

DISRUPTIONS TO A HEALTHY METABOLISM

In the modern world, obesity rates continue to rise. However, those who are clinically overweight or are obese are often frowned upon by others. They are often labeled as being weak-willed or simply lazy. This is not true. For years, the wrong messages about which foods were nutrient rich, healthy, and essential to a standard diet were incorrect. In addition, the growing global availability of junk food and fast food have also exacerbated the obesity problem. Fast food chains are now found in locations that are rich and poor, all over the world. Poor food quality and hidden sugars found in nearly all fast food and processed items are deadly. Cookies, potato chips, and other processed "treats" are a standard staple of nearly everyone's snack preferences and overall diets. It is hard to resist because of its heavy marketing and advertising, affordability, and universal access. All of these factors contribute to this health crisis, which is anchored in metabolic disorders.

The popularity of prescription drugs to treat an unhealthy metabolism often do harm in other ways. Typically, it becomes even more difficult to lose weight because of the chemical properties and hormone effects that mingle in the body. Additionally, weakened immune systems also contribute to difficulties in losing weight and improving health.

The Atkins Diet addresses the correct and most nutrient beneficial foods and attempts to answer why some people struggle to lose weight in the face of these challenges. For one, the availability of these sugar filled foods, heavy consumption, and incorrect knowledge lead to metabolic resistance over time, making it even more difficult for individuals who are overweight or obese to lose weight in order to improve their health.

A healthy metabolism is important for a full and unlimited life. The Atkins Diet can help you restore your health and regain your outlook on what is possible about how you feel. The most important step to take is to inform yourself of what the Atkins Diet is and how it can help (which this guide does!) and to commit to the nutritional approach.

The vast majority of all weight loss problems stem from a weakened metabolism. Excess insulin is found in nearly all overweight and obese individuals. The best solution if to limit refined carbohydrates immediately. There is no nutritional value in food items like potato chips, cookies, or even bread. The incorrect food pyramid has led people down a destructive path all these years by advocating the importance of wheat and grains, which is not true. Proteins, healthy fats, and vegetables are the only vital components needed in a person's diet in order to stay energized. When followed in accordance to the Atkins Diet principles, this is the source of unlimited physical potential.

The role of prescription drugs in causing disruptions in

optimal metabolic functioning should not be overlooked. In today's fast moving modern world, the pharmaceutical industry holds tremendous power. However, lifestyle and improper food guidelines and marketing can cause people to seek out these prescription drugs, which actually prevent individuals from a losing weight.

Birth control pills, diet pills, anti-anxiety or anti-depression medication, insulin injections or pills, and pain killers are incredibley powerful and create an imbalanced interior system. This has numerous effects. It can cause mood swings, food cravings, sickness, and other ailments, which can get in the way of staying on track with the Atkins Diet. The body becomes even more of a challenge. Food cravings and other unhealthy inclinations will be even more difficult to push back against.

Anti-depressants have risen to become the third most popular drug prescribed and used by all Americans today. For extreme mental illnesses and chemical disorders, anti-depressants are an incredibly healing and life-saving medication. However, in today's prescription drug friendly atmosphere, many are over prescribed. There are so many people who do not need this drug. This is dangerous.

Today, popular anti-depressants like Paxil, Prozac, or Zoloft are widely advertised and may be available through a visit to a psychiatrist or mental health professional. A problem with these types of drugs are their frequent overprescription. Regardless of the treatment, it is important to understand the chemical components within these drugs.

Psychotropic medication may cause inner imbalances and most notably, weight gain. Anti-depressants contain serotonin, which works to change the feelings of sadness that characterize depression and other mental illness afflictions. Serotonin is often prescribed in situations involving depression because it is a neurotransmitter. While it can and often does improve mood, it does so at a cost to the rest of the body. For instance, some side effects can include fatigue, constipation, and a subpar metabolic system. These are all dangerous for the optimum health that the Atkins Diet tries to provide.

Due to the seriousness of both psychological and physical health, it is important to discuss your diet plans with both your mental health provider in addition to your general physician. Have them work together to find an alternative (if possible) to reduce your prescription medication for your depression or mental health disorder. If the medication is needed, then follow their direction, but try to commit to the Atkins Diet as much as possible. While mental health medication may provide obstacles, it is very possible to fully adopt the Atkins Diet. Have a support system. Talk to your mental health and health providers. Take your medication as instructed. Implement a firm exercise routine. You will feel better. And in time, the Atkins Diet may boost your mood, so that you may begin to talk to your psychiatrist or mental health provider about decreasing or eliminating your prescription. A healthy life awaits.

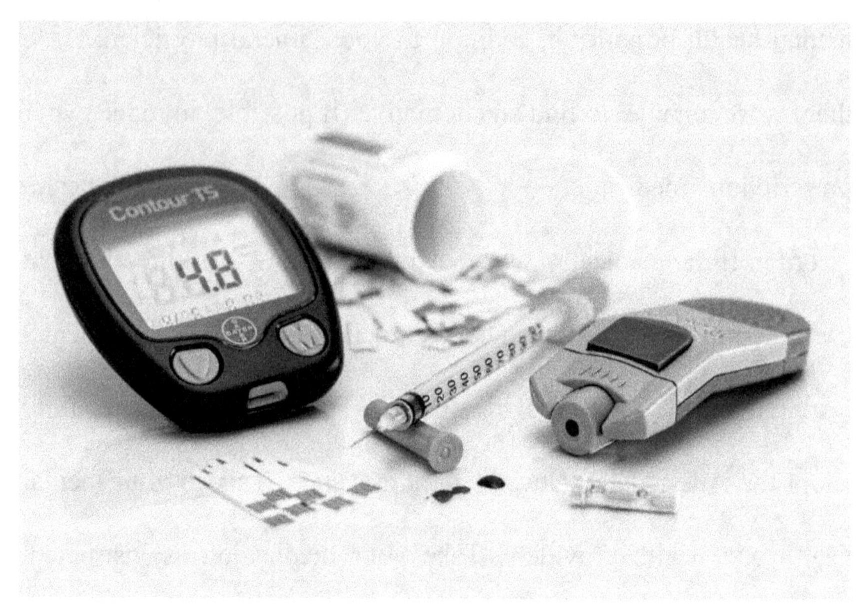

DIABETES AND INSULIN: HOW ATKINS CAN HELP

An unhealthy surplus of insulin in the body from poor eating patterns is common. This usually results in other metabolic resistance difficulties. Excess weight, diabetes, poor functioning, heart disease, cancer, and more can all stem from an unhealthy metabolism.

Diabetes is specifically troubling due to its rapid rise in developed countries. It is a disease where your blood sugar (glucose) levels are dangerously high. In diabetes, your body fails to or has a difficult time making insulin. This is dangerous because every living body needs insulin in order to move glucose to the rest of your interior makeup. If the glucose cannot move through your system and reach your cells, you will begin to have serious health problems. Sadly, these health issues plague many people today. Pre-diabetes or diabetes can lead to stroke and various forms of heart disease, which are leading causes of death today.

Fortunately, with the advancement of technology and information, diabetes can be monitored. Blood work can show existing pre-diabetes or either form of diabetes that exists in the system. The Atkins Diet can help. It aims to helpfully limit the consumption of refined carbohydrates, thus reducing hidden sugars. This, in itself, can help control glucose, while making significant strides towards improving your health for the long-term.

Diabetics are overweight or obese because of their improper levels of insulin. While modern medicine aims to alleviate or lessen the outcome of advanced diabetes, it also affects the system by increasing insulin levels. This makes people more resistant to weight loss, because their metabolism unnaturally changes.

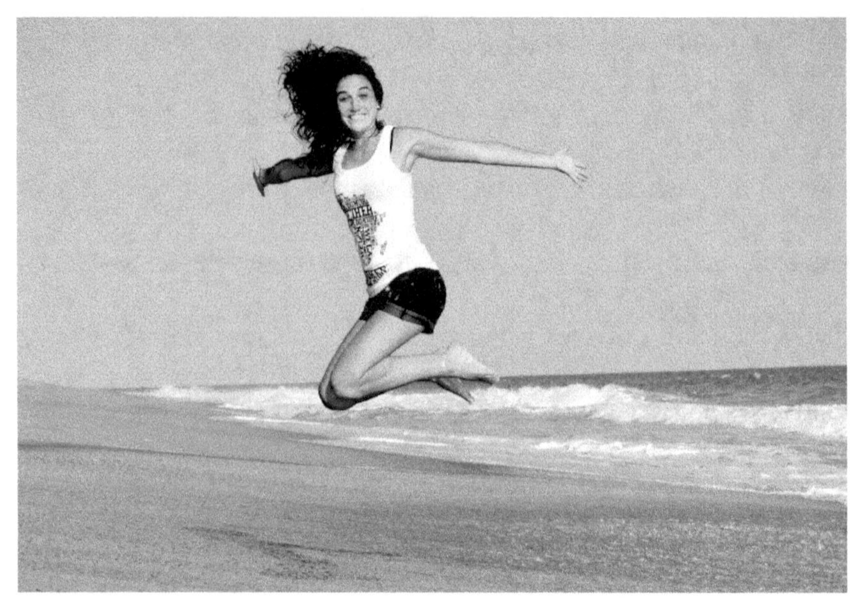

ATKINS DIET SUCCESS

The Atkins Diet has held on to its popularity through the years because its core principles make sense. Its success through both individual accounts and large populations of people are a testament to this. Dr. Atkins' many books on the science and research behind this nutritional approach has continuing sales. This signifies that this diet plan and way of living connects with people.

An unprocessed, high protein diet provides nutrients, energy, and satisfaction. People do not need to overconsume grains and carbohydrates often throughout the day in order to stay full. The

Atkins Diet can supply that full feeling so that people do not use food as a comfort, but instead, learn to view food as it should be—as fuel.

Being an "emotional eater" is a concept that many individuals can relate to. But the Atkins Diet can help. Eating proteins will eliminate the need for excess carbohydrate or fast food consumption. As you will see the weight come off, you will be motivated to continue with what the Atkins Diet can offer you: renewed health. Your weight, metabolic functioning, and outlook on your physicality and overall health will only improve.

Reading food blogs of people's personal weight loss journeys can help motivate you as well. And there are no greater testaments than those who have achieved weight loss success through the Atkins Diet. Numerous personal narratives can show the benefits of committing to the Atkins Diet.

The incorrect, standard diet of many which consists of high carbohydrate consumption and calorie counting is nearly impossible and ineffective. Limiting fat will increase hunger pangs and blood glucose levels defeating the purpose of a nutritional approach, let alone a diet. Cutting sugar, both apparent and hidden, is the key for

health, weight loss, and sustainability.

64

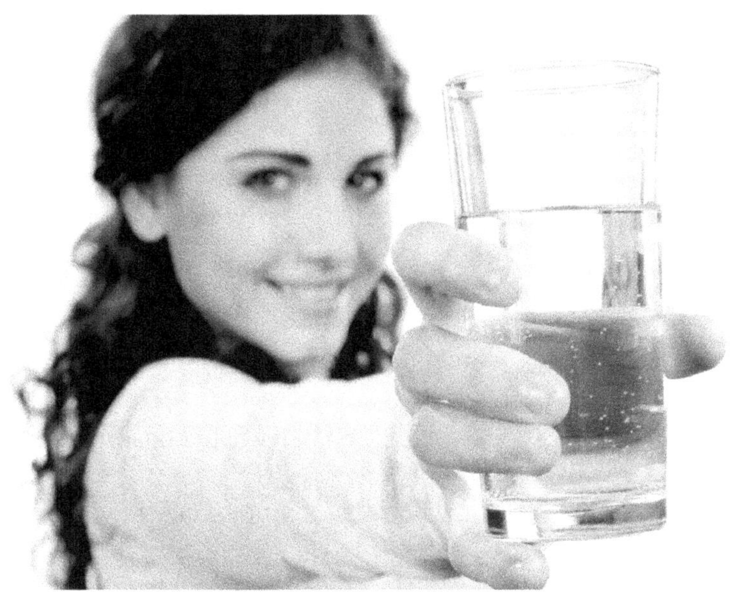

KEYS FOR SUCCESS

When you begin the Induction phase for the Atkins Diet, you may feel overwhelmed. After years of consuming fast food, junk food, grains, pastas, chips, or other staples without much thought or understanding of just how dangerous these foods are, it might be daunting.

The first key to success is to understand what exactly you are consuming right now in your standard, everyday diet. Chances are it's not good. Most likely, you found this book for a reason. And that's because you are wondering how to go about changing your weight, your physical appearance, how you feel, and more.

Give the Atkins Diet a try.

Out of all of the diets that have been written about or that you have decided to check out, the Atkins Diet surpasses them all. It is about eating healthily, not depriving yourself to the point of starvation. Eventually, you will understand what foods your body truly does need. You will learn how much you need to eat in the morning, afternoon, and evening in order to fuel yourself for your job or a specific day. More importantly, you will learn how much or how little you do actually need to eat in order to lose weight.

While it may seem impossible now, you will completely understand how little you need processed and refined carbohydrates like chips or bread. It is standard in the Atkins Diet to follow the Atkins plan, consuming only 20 net carbs per day with varying exceptions in certain cases. However, you may realize that you don't even need those 20 carbs, once you get used to a diet full of protein, healthy fats, and nutritious vegetables. Useless carbohydrates will begin to disappear from your cravings until the day you realize what real food actually is and what good health can do for you.

While many diets claim that their keys for success center around portion control and calorie counting, the Atkins diet tends to rely on common sense and listening to your body. A general guideline would be to have no more than 2,000 calories per day. This varies. It can be slightly less (by about two hundred calories give or take) for women and slightly more (also by about two hundred calories give or take) for men. But the key for success is to eat three (or four smaller) meals per day, with adequate protein in every full meal. Eat until you feel energized, but you should never overeat. Listen to your body and adjust your meal sizes according to your specific physicality.

While the Atkins Diet has its own product line of supplements, shakes, and health bars, you now know what you need to eat based on the information provided in this starter guide. Stick to natural, whole foods. By now, knowing that you should have protein during your three (or four) meals per day should be as natural as reciting your name. Aim for no less than four ounces per regular meal. Lean meats, fish, eggs, and olive oil should be staples in your kitchen.

Fat is not the enemy. Healthy fats are essential in order to feel satisfied nutritionally and so you will consume less food. Healthy fats (never trans fats) are a central component to the Atkins Diet. However, sugar is another story. Cutting out sugar from your diet can improve health, improve or minimize diabetes, and help weight loss. Today, sugar is hidden everywhere. From the obvious like cupcakes, cookies, and other sweets to the less obvious like store salad dressings, potato chips, and other snacks, these line the shelves—sugar is everywhere. So much so, that your daily consumption of it is much higher than you are aware of.

Another crucial key for success is to eat vegetables. Based on the Atkins plan, it is important to eat at least twelve grams of vegetables every day. This is important not only for weight loss, but for energy and excellent health. Vegetables contain plenty of fiber. This regulates blood sugar and sets your system up on a good schedule. The fiber in vegetables (like proteins) leave you feeling satisfied and energized. When you consume refined carbohydrates like pizza, pasta, or junk food for lunch you will often feel sleepy after. This is responsible for that midday crash that many report to feel at work. And you do not want to be sleeping at work!

There are fewer foods that are as nutrient rich, protective, and unquestionably healthy as vegetables. If you have bad memories from childhood from being forced to eat certain vegetables or have a general dislike of certain vegetables, then don't eat those specific ones. There are plenty vegetables to choose from, more than you are aware. So, hit the vegetable aisle at your grocery store or health food store and get familiar. Try new ones! Experiment! And continue to eat the vegetables that you like and can incorporate into your Atkins Diet plan. Regular vegetable consumption is a necessary key for health success and improvement!

In the beginning, it might be helpful to plan meals and snacks for work and outings and to eat at home during off hours. During the Induction phase, this can help to limit temptation from a rushed day, a lack of options, or cravings. Take the necessary steps during the initial phase so that you are nourished and never scrambling to find something to eat. Typically, this will lead to bingeing or an inclination to eat fast food or a meal with nutrient empty carbohydrates.

Another key for success is to drink water after each meal. The Atkins Diet does not allow soft drinks, sugary teas, or artificial juices whatsoever. Water will be your main staple. You will feel good and lose weight. When you follow this key, you will be one step closer to success. You will be one step closer to finding the health, ability, and physicality you have always wanted.

Vitamins and supplements can be helpful. This may be needed, especially after a life full of unhealthy living and a nutrient empty diet. Whole vitamins including vitamin A and D, as well as potassium, calcium, and fish oil can help restore health during this transitional time.

Additionally, exercise is crucial. If you do not like running, try biking. If you are starting out and are overweight and obese, start small. Walking, swimming, yoga, or meditation may help to initiate blood flow and stay centered and committed during the Induction phase, in addition to losing weight. You will begin to feel the change. Once you continue, you won't look back. This is part of your new life…and your success.

Previously, we mentioned how personal food blogs can be

inspirational and motivational. Many out there on the Internet have chronicled their ups and downs on their Atkins weight loss journey. Not only does is signify what might wait ahead for you, it also means that you are part of a strong community. Personal online food diaries are symbols and accounts of people who are committed to change and are bettering themselves. It does not happen in a day or two days. It is a journey and a life change. Chronicle your story. Share it with others. Inspire others to research the Atkins Diet and to read this book and others.

If the online blog world is too intimidating, then keep a private diary. Chronicle your victories. Congratulate yourself on paper and with your support system when you follow the Atkins Diet guidelines. Write down how you feel. Journaling honestly can push your further towards your goal and can keep you living this way. Once you feel this good, you will never want to go back to the way things were, or how you felt back then.

Your other support system should be a trusted individual or a trusted group of friends. Trusted is the key word. Negative people surround all of us whether we like it or not. This is another time when it is important to be selective. So, if you have a critical person in your life who stirs up toxic feelings, try to keep your distance from them during this time. And make the decision *not* to share your diet plan with them. They may derail your success and your commitment to Atkins even after you've succeeded, which you will!

Much like sharing your Atkins Diet journey through a blog, sharing your Atkins success with a trusted individual or small group may inspire them to do the same. And this is one of the benefits of committing to a diet plan as sensible and energizing as the Atkins Diet. So be proud of how far you've come and enjoy your much-deserved success. By sheer will, determination, and commitment, you have found the nutritional approach that will shape your life for the better! Congratulations! Now let's continue on!

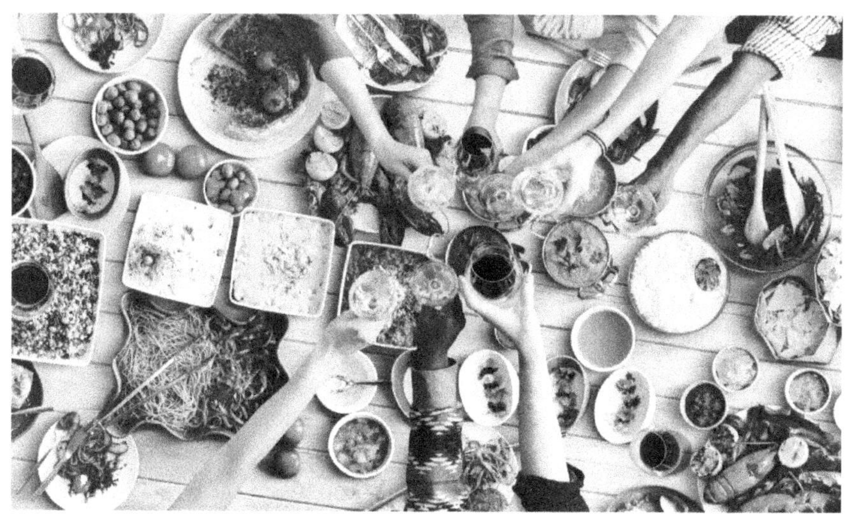

THE ATKINS DIET IS FOR EVERYONE

All adults fall victim to stress, extenuating life circumstances, or other obstacles which can lead to difficult times. Often these problematic periods can lead to a dependence or an inclination to alleviate or mask pain. Many people fall prey to the temporary fixes that alcohol, drugs, and more commonly food can provide. However, it is only a temporary fix. In the long-term, it will not solve anything. It will only make things worse. But only you can fix your life and your health.

You are not alone. Large portions of the population have a carbohydrate addiction and consequently, a metabolic disorder. And many people get drastic. They begin to starve and exercise themselves to death, often avoiding fat, and eat as little as possible. This will always lead to overeating at a later time.

A low carb diet and healthy proteins and vegetables will lead to a good place. You can eat to fill nourished, energized, and happy! And once you complete the phases of the Atkins Diet, you will not have to monitor grams or restrict fruit, because you will know what is right for you and how to practice self-control.

Starving yourself is never the answer. Nor is counting calories. That is not the way to live. To make a lasting, permanent change you have to fuel your body, so you can handle whatever other life stressors come in your way.

You can eradicate two to three pounds every two weeks just from cutting out processed carbohydrates from your diet. What's even better is when you realize that you don't need them. Food should be fuel. This is what the Atkins Diet helps you understand that by nourishing your body you are fueling it for life.

During the Induction phase, the weight loss can be your motivator. Seeing the pounds continue to vanish can further your cause. But the thing that will sustain you on this journey is the fact that these new foods are satisfying and filling. No more mindless snacking. No more pizza binges after a day of calorie counting. This is not what the Atkins Diet promotes. For each individual, the Atkins Diet can help you look at food through a new perspective. You will no longer zero in on the pizza without remembering how bloated and heavy it made you feel after. You will no longer look at the burger without remembering how sleepy it made you in the middle of the day at work. You will remember how heavy you used to be, how sluggish, and how sad at how you could not participate in certain activities out of fear, insecurity, or sheer inability. Those days are over. Your new life has begun! Don't wait! With this book, you can move forward today and every day. There is nothing stopping you now.

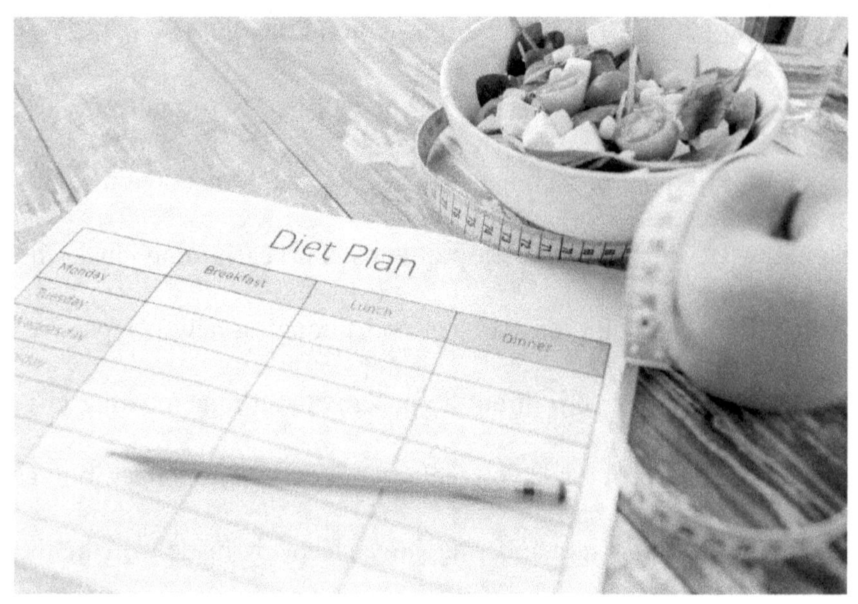

SAMPLE ATKINS DIET MEAL PLANS

Breakfast might include:

- Two small lean turkey patties and a few mushrooms or

- Two scrambled egg whites and sundried tomatoes

Lunch:

- Small serving of a chicken breast with lemon juice on top or

- Green leafy salad with olives, feta cheese, and tomato

Snack (or smaller meal):

- Celery sticks and tuna

- Carrot sticks dipped in vinegar and olive oil

- Diced tomato drizzled with olive oil and a sprinkle of salt

Dinner:

- Cooked Portobello mushrooms

- Beef cooked in olive oil with onions

- A few asparagus seasoned with salt, pepper, tarragon, lemon, or olive oil

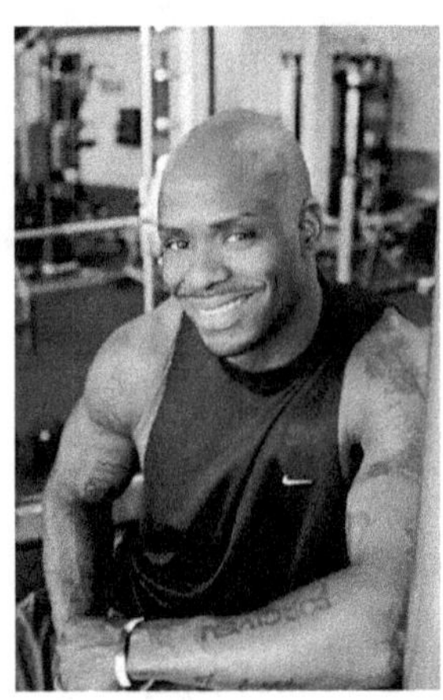

ABOUT THE AUTHOR

Hello, my name is Justin!

I hope you like my books. Let me tell you a little about myself.

For 7 years now I have been working as a personal fitness trainer.

During this time, I realized that it is not enough just to make an effective training plan. Training in the hall is only a small part of the work on the way to a healthy, strong and beautiful body. In my opinion, the formula looks like this: 30% training, 30% an active way of life and positive thinking, and 40% healthy eating.

I like to cook, I love to write, and I like to invent recipes. All my knowledge and passion were embodied in my books.

There is a huge variety of diets that allow you to quickly lose weight. I'm not sure they are all useful. In my books, I write about diets that not only lead to weight loss, but also give health and vivacity. I hope they will benefit you, too!

Be sure to subscribe to the newsletter to receive news of new books and bonuses from me.

With love,

Justin